<u>Dr. Anna Steve.</u>

H -PYLORI

TREATMENT.

With a 7-Day diet plan.

A Healing Guide to Peptic Ulcer, Idiopathic Thrombocytopenic Purpura (ITP), Mood Swings, Heart Related Diseases, Dyspepsia, Hormonal Imbalance, Colorectal Cancer, Lymphomas, Pregnancy Related Infections. *ENT (Ear, Nose And Throat), Liver And Gall-Bladder Illness, Pulmonary Disease, Tuberculosis, Bronchiectasis & Inflammatory Bowel Disease (IBD), Central Serous Retinopathy (CSR) And Ocular (Eye) Diseases, etc.*

H -PYLORI TREATMENT.

This book has been independently written and published strictly for informational and educational purpose(s) only.   It is not intended to serve as a medical prescription of any kind. You should endeavor to consult/visit a professional healthcare expert before embarking on any medical or dietary therapy.

This book or any portion thereof may not reproduced or used in any manner whatsoever, without due recourse to the publisher.

Foreword.

…the helicobacter pylori is a bacterial that is so underrated and little is known about. It is the primary cause of peptic ulcer, associated with the stomach lining. This book by Dr. Anna is an eye-opener to H-pylori, how to treat is, and all about ulcer.

… Dr. Emily Clifford.
(MD) *former Westwood Clinic Physician, TX.*

Table of Contents.

H -PYLORI TREATMENT.

H -PYLORI TREATMENT.

H -PYLORI TREATMENT.

CHAPTER ONE.

INTRODUCTION TO HELICOBACTER PYLORI (H-PYLORI).

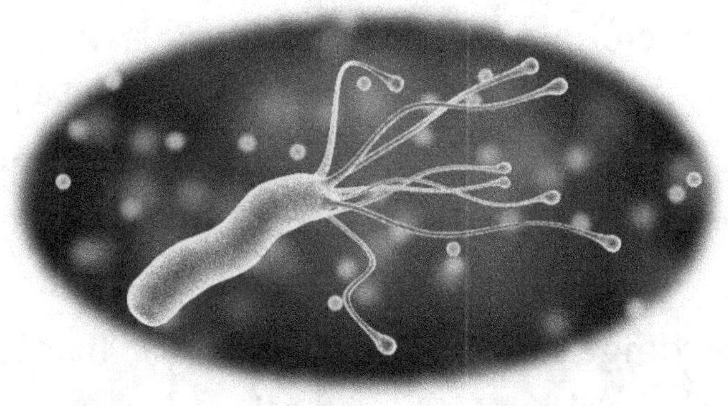

Before now, humanity has been greatly affected by the persistent and distressing existence of the H-pylori bacterium in the human body, which leads to peptic ulcer, but it was thought to be as a result of stress and unattended anxiety-related disorders.

However, thousands of years ago, two scientists Marshall and Warren discovered the leading cause of the peptic ulcer to be the Helicobacter pylori bacteria. It is the first bacteria to be identified as a leading cause of stomach cancer. Infact, the IARC categorized this H-pylori bacteria as group 1 in the categorization of cancer-causing agents.

According to research, H-pylori bacteria make up about 20% of all cancer-related illnesses around the globe.

WHAT IS HELICOBACTER PYLORI?

Helicobacter pylori also known as H-pylori is a kind of bacteria that is recognised to infect the stomach. This bacterium is seldomly known as the brain behind inflammatory and sore-related injuries in the stomach's walls/lining. H-pylori also goes as far as affecting the small intestine, and digestive tracts of some persons and when not swiftly attended to, could further cascade to stomach-related cancerous growth.

According to research, millions of persons around the globe have H -pylori within their body system, and its related infections are very common. Studies have also shown that it doesn't exhibit any symptom(s) for most persons. It can also result in peptic ulcer.

Helicobacter Pylori (H-pylori) could also be called a pathogen which could alter the immunity response and physiological characteristics of their hosts. H-pylori is a cause of death for over 65,000 persons around the globe annually.

Other species of H-pylori:

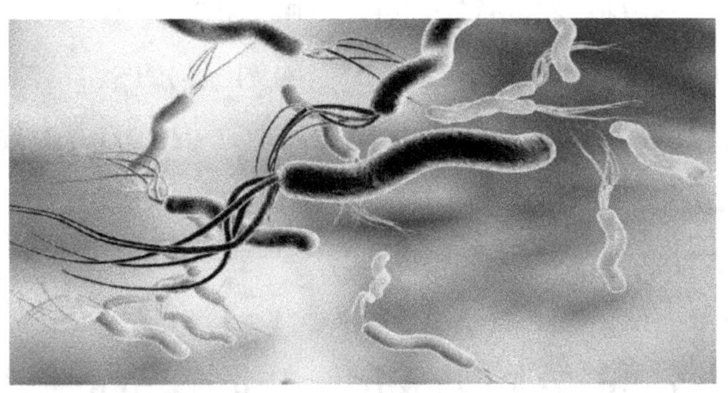

Although more medical research is still ongoing, it has been proven that there are some other notable species of H-pylori, that colonize other parts of the body other than the stomach. Some of these species include;

H- cinaedi, H- Canis, H- Fennelliae, H- Billis, H- Hepaticus, H-Suis, H- Rappini, H- Pullorum, H- Heilmannii, H- Salmonis, H- Bizzozeronii, H- Canadensis and others.

CHAPTER TWO.

ULCER, AND ITS TYPES.

Simply put, an ulcer is a painful wound or sole that commonly happens within the stomach or belly region, creating a hole/cavity and its healing process is very slow. Outside the stomach, ulcers can occur in any part of the body, and in most cases, they require the attention of a medical health professional.

<u>TYPES OF ULCERS:</u>

There are basically four (4) types of ulcers, viz-a-viz;

- ↳ *Genital ulcers*
- ↳ *Mouth ulcers*
- ↳ *Arterial (ischemic) ulcers and,*
- ↳ *Venous ulcers.*
- ↳ **<u>ARTERIAL ULCERS:</u>**

Arterial ulcer which is also known by the name ischemic ulcer. It is an open sore that is inside the miniature side of the capillaries and arterioles, notably around the leg area, and it is prevalent in individuals who have low blood pressure.

This is another type of ulcer that also affects the leg, ankle, and foot region of the body. This venous is not associated with pain as such, not except when they are infected. If infected can be very painful as well and they take a long time to heal. A certified health professional should be contacted in the treatment of this kind of ulcer.

⇘ MOUTH ULCERS:

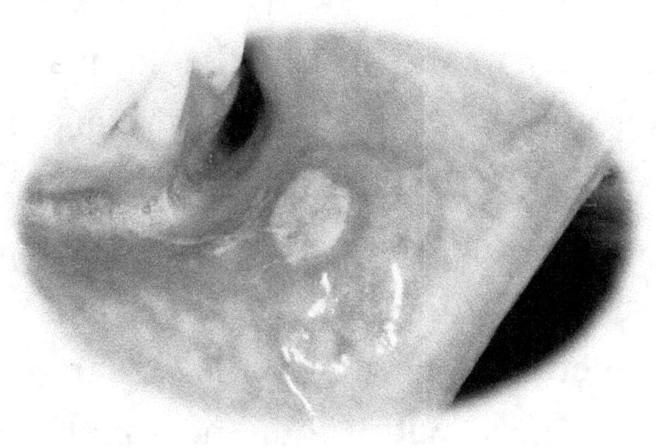

These are ulcer types that develop in the mouth and the gum area. They happen as small sores, and they are normally triggered by a number of risk factors such as hormonal change, bacteria infection, vitamin deficiencies, stress, and others.

When medically attended to, they are treated within 7-14 days but can develop into serious wounds when left untreated.

⮑ <u>GENITAL ULCERS:</u>

These types of ulcers are found around the genital region of the body. They are sores that develop in and around the vagina, anus, and scrotum, and are sexually transmitted, however, in other situations, they can be induced by other diseases like inflammation and traumatic conditions.

This ulcer type normally disappears on its own. Discuss with your personal health expert when you have such an ulcer condition.

CHAPTER THREE.

PEPTIC ULCER & H-PYLORI.

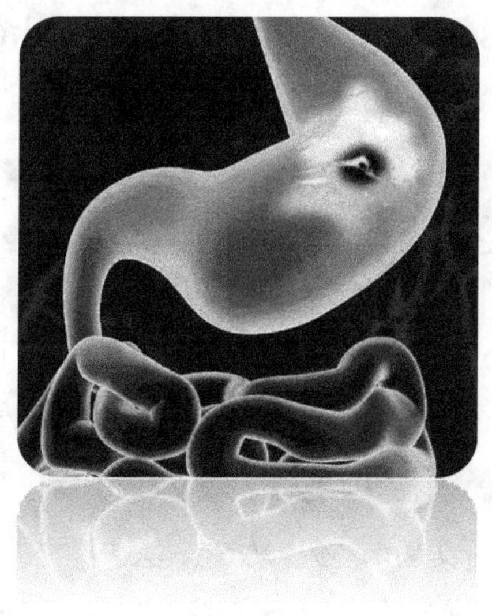

Peptic ulcers are open wounds or sores in the wall-lining of the stomach. They can also appear in the esophagus and small intestine area or region of the stomach. Research has shown that they are caused mainly by inflammation resulting from the presence of Helicobacter pylori, commonly known as H-pylori. Peptic ulcers could also result due to the presence of excessive acidic content in the stomach.

<u>TYPES OF PEPTIC ULCERS.</u>

For the purpose of this book, there are basically three types of known peptic ulcers. They include;

- *The Gastric peptic ulcer,*
- *The Duodenal peptic ulcer and*
- *The Esophageal peptic ulcer.*

➥ <u>**THE GASTRIC PEPTIC ULCER.**</u>

Just in tandem with the nomenclature, the gastric peptic ulcer is/are commonly found in the stomach wall lining of the human body. They are also caused by the excessive presence of acidic content in the body, as well as H-pylori bacteria.

➥ <u>**THE ESOPHAGEAL PEPTIC ULCER.**</u>

This type or kind of ulcer mainly occurs in the wall lining region of the esophagus. It is caused mainly by the H-pylori bacteria.

➥ <u>**THE DUODENAL PEPTIC ULCERS.**</u>

This peptic ulcer type normally occurs or develops in the small intestine. The top region of the small intestine is where this ulcer is largely felt. This part of the human body is commonly known as the duodenum.

Every infection, ailment, or disease has its cause, and so does the peptic ulcer infection. For a quick glance, below are some of the possible peptic ulcer causes;

- *H-pylori bacteria,*
- *Excessive smoking,*
- *Exposure to radiation,*
- *Alcoholism,*

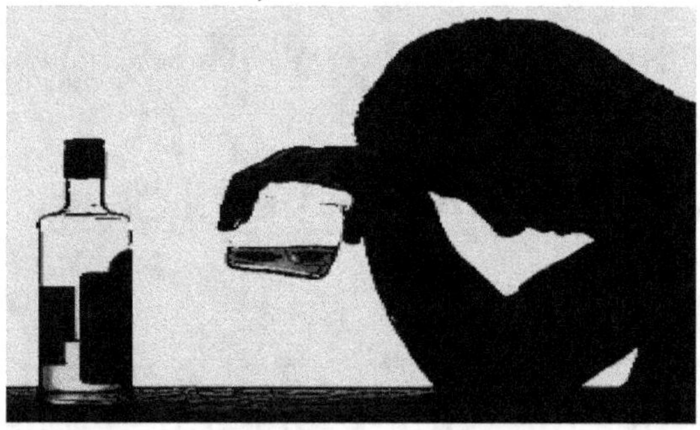

- *Stomach-related cancer and abusive use of ibuprofen and aspirin drugs.*

POSSIBLE SYMPTOMS OF PEPTIC ULCER.

When you happen to have a peptic ulcer, below are some possible symptoms that might exhibit, viz-a-viz;

- *Blood-stained faeces,*
- *Nausea and vomiting,*

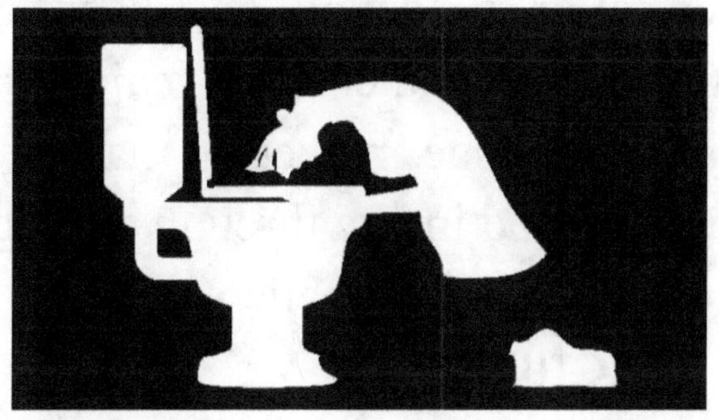

- *Constipation,*
- *Unstable appetite,*
- *Weight loss as well as consistent stomach upset.*

POSSIBLE COMPLICATIONS OF THE PEPTIC ULCER ILLNESS.

When left unattended, peptic ulcers could lead to some more deadly resultant effects. Some of these may include;

- **<u>SCAR TISSUE:</u>**

Scars are known to be tissues that are created after a wound has been healed. Regardless of whether it is a major or minor injury, the tissue makes it hard for the passage of food intake through the digestive tract of a peptic ulcer patient.

- **<u>PUNCTURE:</u>**

The peptic ulcer creates a kind of cavity in the wall lining of the stomach and small intestine. This could lead to very severe pain in the abdominal region of the stomach.

- **<u>INTERNAL INJURY:</u>**

Internal injury which will lead to bleeding, could result in a very significant loss of blood, faintness, and when not treated on time, could result to death. Medical consultations should be made before further actions are carried out.

<u>CHAPTER FOUR.</u>

<u>CONTRACTING, DIAGNOSING & TESTING HELICOBACTER-PYLORI.</u>

H-pylori is a bacteria and it is contagious from one individual to the other. It is highly contaminable through water, unsterilized utensils, and the exchange of bodily fluids.

POSSIBLE RISK FACTORS THAT COULD CAUSE H -PYLORI.

From research, whether you are an adult or an infant, you can contract H -pylori, but kids are most susceptible/vulnerable. Some of these risk factors include but are not limited to the following:

- *Lack of social distancing.*
- *Drinking of unhygienic water*
- *Living with someone who has H-pylori without adequate health safety.*

POSSIBLE SYMPTOMS OF H -H-PYLORI.

There are some possible signs that could be traced to the H -pylori infection. They include;

- *Feeling a burning sensation in the belly*
- *Belching,*
- *Stomach bloating/inflammation*
- *Nausea and vomiting and some kind of bodily weight loss.*

<u>WHAT DOES H-PYLORI SUFFERERS' POOP LOOK LIKE?</u>

There are some misconceptions as to the look of the excreta of a person that is infected by H -pylori. The faeces of an infected person don't look abnormal in any way, when your excreta become too black, or has some blood stains, it is expedient that you contact the services of your health care practitioner.

Other symptoms that may result in you contacting your healthcare expert include viz-a-viz;

- *Continuous feeling of dizziness,*
- *Paleness of skin,*
- *Difficulty in breathing,*
- *Persistent vomiting of black substances,*
- *Continuous and persistent sharp sensation around the stomach.*

DIAGNOSING H-PYLORI.

The testing for H-pylori presence is/are grouped into two categories: The invasive method and the non-invasive method.

INVASIVE TEST:

The Urea breath method of testing encompasses the drinking of both Carbons

(C-13 and C-14) radiolabelled urea samples. The intake of carbon is then converted to carbon-dioxide and NH3 (Ammonia) as a result of the presence of urea. This carbon-dioxide is then taken to the lab and analyzed for the presence of the hitherto ingested labeled carbon. This breath test is by far the most sensitive and highly efficient test for H-pylori antigens presence with over 98% true result.

NON-INVASIVE TEST:

According to researchers, the sensitivity and trueness of this test is about 90%. It is a more economical method of testing.

- **THE SEROLOGY TESTING METHOD:**

In this test, microtiter plates are provided with embedded H-pylori antigens. This testing procedure is easily accessible and very cost-effective. It is worthy of note that the serology process or procedure does not confirm the eradication of H-pylori, and it doesn't validate the up-to-date state of H-pylori infection in the body. The sensitivity and trueness of this testing procedure are just above 80%.

From research, it has been ascertained that there are some ways to diagnose H -pylori-related infection. Some of these diagnosing processes include;

⇛ <u>THE STOOL ANTIGEN TEST:</u>

This is a simple and the most conventional test of trying to detect the presence of proteinous antigens in the defecation of a suspected sufferer of H-pylori.

↳ **THE PCR FAECES TEST:**

Also known as the Polymerase Chain Reaction test, the PCR stool test watches out for any possible way of mutations for antibiotic-resistant bacteria, but this test is more expensive than the formal.

↳ **THE UREA BREATH TEST:**

To begin this test, get a doctor's bag and get yourself to exhale your breath into the bag (your carbon dioxide breath). After this first exhale of your breath, swallow your urea pudding as provided by your health practitioner, wait for about 10 to 20 minutes, and then exhale/breathe out carbon dioxide in another bag.

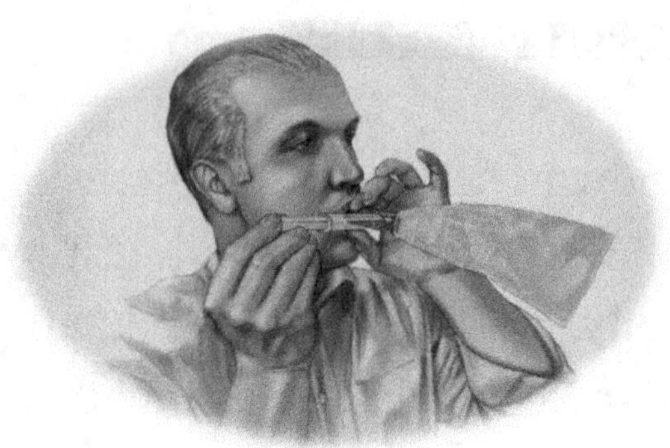

These bags with the exhale samples are then sent to a laboratory for test comparison. When you happen to have H - pylori in your gut system, it will break down the urea substance in the pudding that you took in and CO_2 will be released. Also, if there happens to be more CO_2 present in the last bag breath sample than it is in the first, then your test for H -pylori presence is positive.

➥ <u>**THE UPPER GASTROINTESTINAL ENDOSCOPY TEST:**</u>

In carrying out this test, your health practitioner will use a tube attached to an endoscopic camera to take a look at the inside of your throat, down your stomach, and small intestine.

This tube attached to an endoscope can be used to collect some bodily fluid samples that will be tested for H -pylori.

⇨ THE UPPER G.I TESTS:

With the help of your health care expert, barium (whitish chalky liquid) will be swallowed. The substance will be seen to cover or coat the walls of your throat and stomach.

⇨ THE CT SCAN TEST:

The computed Tomography (CT) scan is an X-ray-related scan that is used to detect the potential condition or state of your peptic ulcers in the stomach.

CHAPTER FIVE.

HELICOBACTER PYLORI PROPERTIES, COMPLICATIONS, & PREVENTIONS.

Helicobacter pylori (H-pylori) is a heterogenous morphological microaerophilic bacteria that strives in an atmospheric temperature of 10% carbon-dioxide and 5% oxygen.

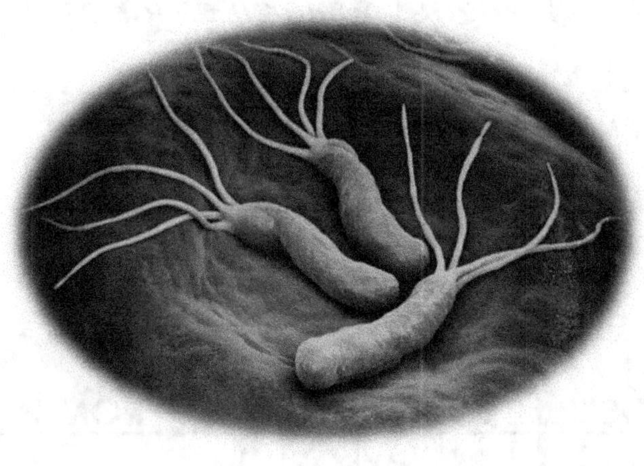

Morphology	Heterogenous
Atmospheric conditions to strive	*10% carbondioxide and 5% oxygen.*
Shape	*Helicoidal, and spiral*
Numbers of Flagella	*Ranges from 2 to 7*
Diameter	*From 0.5mm to 1.0mm*
Overall length	*Some go as far as 5mm long.*
Incubation period	*4 to 5 days*

POSSIBLE COMPLICATIONS FROM H-PYLORI.

This ailment can result in inflammatory-related discomfort, vomiting, and nausea.

When the ailment is left unattended to per treatment, it could lead to some health-related complications, such as;

- *Bleeding in the stomach.*
- *Cavity hole in your stomach wall.*
- *Acute constipation.*

<u>PREVENTING H -H-PYLORI.</u>

Just like every disease or illness, there are preventions and cures when properly managed. H-pylori is not an exception to this as it is as the popular saying goes that a stitch in time saves nine.

Some of the known ways to prevent you from contracting the H-pylori infection is to avoid bacteria contact through the following ways;

- *Practice good hygiene*
- *Encourage those around you to practice good and safe hygiene*

- *Ensure you eat well-cooked meals*
- *Drink clean water and avoid unhealthy living conditions.*

WHAT YOUR HEALTH CARE PROVIDER SHOULD CONSIDER BEFORE TREATING YOU FROM H-PYLORI.

When you meet your medical professional expert to help with your treating the H-pylori bacteria infection, your medical expert should consider the following;

- *The seriousness of the infection case,*
- *Your age group,*
- *Past and overall health history/condition,*
- *Your past response to certain medications, and treatment.*

PEOPLE WHO ARE MAINLY AT RISK OF CONTRACTING H-PYLORI.

Just like every other infection, H-pylori has a group of individuals who are considered as those mainly at risk of contracting the bacteria infection. They include;

- ## **<u>Age Group:</u>**

According to research individuals who are 50-years and above are most prone to contracting this bacteria infection.

- ## **<u>Family Traits:</u>**

When you happen to have traits of bacterial infection in your immediate family, you might be prone to contracting the H-pylori infection.

<u>H -PYLORI INFECTION IN CHILDREN.</u>

Helicobacter pylori apart from affecting adults, also affects infants and children who are exposed to bacteria. The most noticeable symptom of H-pylori in children is gastritis in the stomach.

Reach out to your health expert if your child or ward shows signs of sudden or sharp abdominal pains, blood-stained related faeces, or incessant vomiting.

PREPARING TO VISIT A DOCTOR.

If you happen to have any of the symptoms highlighted above and you schedule a visit to your healthcare provider, below are some of the things that you should do before or during such visit;

- *First and most importantly, write out possible questions that you would like to ask the health expert.*

- *If you happen to be unable to write and speak well, take someone along with you who can help you out with the questions.*

- *When possible, write out the treatment patterns, medications, and other instructions that you were given by your doctor.*

- *Except otherwise stated, always try to write down the date of the next appointment.*

- *Ask for the contact of your health care expert, which should need to be for you to ask further questions or make inquiries after you have left there.*

CHAPTER SIX.

SOME DISEASES/ILLNESSES TREATED BY HELICOBACTER PYLORI.

⇨ H-Pylori And Mood Swings.

Medical and scientific research has it that H-pylori is extensively interconnected with mental and brain functions. The bacteria infection if not well treated could have a resultant depressional and anxiety-related mental breakdown in the carrier.

⇨ H-Pylori And The Heart.

The Helicobacter Pylori infection has been traced in recent research to have some cardiovascular effects on its carrier. H-pylori is known to stimulate the rise of triglyceride and cholesterol but will result in a decline in the HDL 7, 24 cholesterol that will lead to dyslipidemia which is a cardiovascular threat.

✎ Hormonal Imbalance And H -Pylori.

A hormonal imbalance could be stimulated by variance in cortisol, dopamine, and serotonin (5-HT) levels, in the circulatory system, with resultant harm to the CNS (Central Nervous System) in the human body

✎ H-Pylori And Atmospheric Oxygen.

Research has it that the helicobacter pylori bacteria is microaerophilic, that is it cannot live outside the host's body. It dies when exposed to atmospheric oxygen, ambient oxygen, and phagocytic blood cells.

⇝ H- Pylori, Dyspepsia, And Ulcers.

Pain that is relatively associated with the upper abdomen and the stomach is known as dyspepsia. Ulcers also lead to dyspepsia. Proven evidence has some traces that H-pylori disease influences the cases of dyspepsia-related infection.

⇝ H -Pylori And Gastric Cancer.

H-pylori has been established as a root/known cause of Gastric Adenocarcinoma and MALT lymphoma. This kind of cancerous growth is split into two, namely; diffuse and intestinal.

The intestinal gastric adenocarcinoma is the most conventional and most talked about subtype. Researchers have come to the conclusion that incessant smoking, is a major risk factor for this gastric cancer type.

Studies have shown that the transformations made are pathological, and these occur over a long span of years, which leads to an intestinal can type, beginning with gastritis, then the atrophical gastric, and then to intestinal metaplasia, closely followed by dysplasia and carcinoma. This cancer type is age-related.

However, the diffuse type of gastric adenocarcinoma is epitomized and flung by cancerous cells. Helicobacter pylori infection brings about the hypermethylation of the gene encoding E-cadherin. This type of cancer is mostly associated with juvenile and middle-aged individuals.

⮑ <u>H-Pylori And Colorectal Cancer.</u>

This malignant growth type is a form of extragastric cancer that is greatly induced by the presence of H-pylori in colorectal adenocarcinoma.

A study was conducted on patients who are host to some malignant growth like Hyperplastic Ademona, colon, and advanced adenoma as well as colon cancer-related diseases, for the presence of H-pylori in each of them, it was revealed from test result analysis from the laboratory, that the colon cancer had the highest trace of H-pylori.

✎ H -Pylori And Lymphomas.

Studies have shown that the presence of H-pylori increases the risk of lymphoma cancer type. It is not the same as *gastric MALT lymphoma.* DLBCL (Diffuse Large B-cell Lymphoma) is a type of cancerous growth that majorly occurs in the belly region.

✎ H-Pylori And Idiopathic Thrombocytopenic Purpura (ITP).

ITP is closely associated with the destruction of autoimmune platelets, causing significant harm to the body. Studies show that H-pylori is the leading cause of this, as when the H-pylori infection was treated in affected persons, their platelet levels increased tremendously.

⇨ H-Pylori And Skin-Related Infections.

Samples of patients suffering from rosacea skin infection were taken to the laboratory for testing and over 80% of the patients tested positive for the presence of H-pylori. Rosacea is an inflammatory skin infection that can transcend to chronic prurigo, which is an intense itching sensation on the skin.

⇨ H- Pylori And Pregnancy Related Infections.

A recent study shows that about 80% of hyperemesis gravidarum patients (a pregnancy condition that influences protracted vomiting) when their samples were taken for laboratory tests, showed a positive presence of H-pylori bacteria in them.

> ✍ **H-Pylori And The ENT (Ear, Nose And Throat).**

The esophagus and oral cavity of the body are some of the places where H-pylori can be found in the human body. The ear, nose, and throat are all intertwined parts of the gastroesophageal region of the body.

Studies have shown that H-pylori was present in the middle ears of some patients who suffer from tympanosclerosis or otitis medium, when the *Campylobacter*-Like Organism test (CLO) was used to check.

Another study reviewed that there is an inverse correlation between esophageal adenocarcinoma disease and helicobacter pylori infection. That means that, when there is an increase in the prevalence of H-pylori infection in the ENT regions, there would be a decrease in esophageal-related illnesses.

🗦 <u>H- Pylori For Liver And Gall-Bladder Illness.</u>

Researchers have discovered a correlation between H- pylori presence in gallbladder and liver infections in humans. Patients suffering from hepatocellular carcinoma in livers.

Also, sufferers of cholecystitis whose samples were tested showed the presence of H-pylori in their gallbladder mucosa with a high level of inducible nitric oxide synthase, metaplasia, and adenomyomatosis

✎ **<u>H-Pylori And Pulmonary Disease, Tuberculosis, Bronchiectasis & Inflammatory Bowel Disease (IBD).</u>**

Some research has shown the presence of H-pylori infection in Chronic Obstructive Pulmonary Disease (COPD) and bronchiectasis diseases. A group of COP, IBD, TB, and bronchiectasis patients were examined, and the result showed over 50% positivity to the presence of the helicobacter pylori infection.

✎ **<u>H-Pylori On Central Serous Retinopathy (CSR) And Ocular (Eye) Diseases.</u>**

Ocular-related diseases are those diseases that are in relation to the eyes. H-pylori infection has been traced to be a cause of some eye infections, such as glaucoma. In one of the recent studies, patients with ocular diseases were found to be recovering more and getting better when H-pylori eradication therapy was conducted.

✍ <u>H- Pylori, Gastric Ghrelin And Diabetes.</u>

The presence of H-pylori infection in the production of ghrelin compounds suppresses the gastric ghrelin levels in the stomach. From a study, it was discovered that there was a noticeable rise/upsurge in the level of ghrelin presence when H-pylori was eradicated.

✍ <u>H-Pylori, NMO And Multiple Sclerosis Diseases.</u>

Research has shown the presence of H-pylori infection in the delayed recovery of sufferers of Multiple Sclerosis Disease, and Neuromyelitis Optica (NMO). Neuromyelitis Optica disease is known to be an autoimmune infection where some antibodies are in opposition to aquaporin, thereby leading to a demyelination of the optic nerve and spinal cord system of the body. If not promptly addressed, this could result in blindness and complete paralysis of the host.

CHAPTER SEVEN.

RECOMMENDED FOODS TO EAT AND NOT-TO-EAT, WITH H-PYLORI.

Here are some recommended food types that are healthy for consumption for an individual with H-pylori.

➻ **MANUKA HONEY:**

This is a special kind of honey that is produced by bees that pollinate inherent tea trees.

This tree has some good natural antibiotic characteristics. Manuka honey has a great deal of antibacterial features that help to fight against the effect of H-pylori. Research has shown that the consumption of this honey has helped in no small way to reduce the bacteria from the stomach lining of individuals who have gastritis. This honey can be added to your tea, coffee or corn-pap.

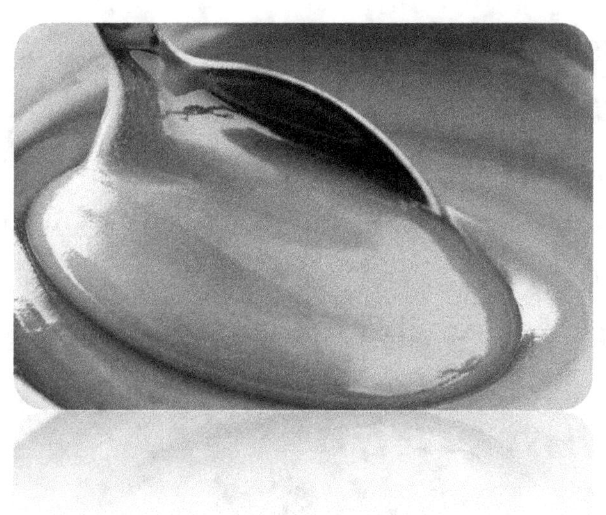

⇨ **<u>FRUITS AND VEGGIES:</u>**

Consumption of healthy non-acidic fruits like cranberries, strawberries, and raspberries is recommended due to the fact that they are quick to digest and improve bowel function in the body.

⇨ **<u>FOODS THAT CONTAINS OMEGA-3 AND OMEGA-6 ACIDS:</u>**

Foods such as fish, pure veggie oils, and carrots and its seed, with omega-3 and 6 acids, have been proven or known to reduce the negative effect of stomach inflammation and to prevent the unhealthy growth of the Helicobacter pylori infection in the body.

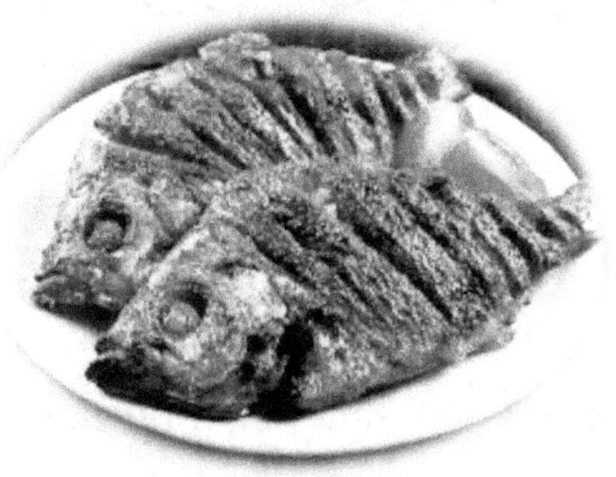

⇘ **<u>PROBIOTICS:</u>**

Infact, this is one of the major nutritional constituents that is found in yoghurt and kefir drinks. Probiotics or their supplements help to stimulate the small intestine for the secretion of a substance called flora, which is proven to be an effective depressant for Helicobacter pylori disease and as such, helps to lower the potential side effects that may tend to occur during treatment from the H-pylori bacteria infection.

✑ <u>**THE CRANBERRIES FRUIT:**</u>

These fruits are well known for their being predominantly antioxidants. If you can't have access to the natural fruits, the extracted capsules, syrup or its medically fit alternative could be used to eradicate or greatly inhibit the growth of the H-pylori infection. About 200-220mls polyphenol, when administered twice a day for one week, has proven to reduce the helicobacter pylori effect.

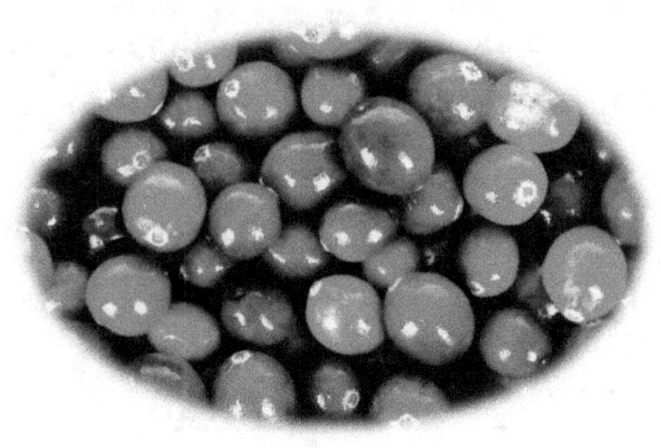

⇘ **THE BLACK CUMIN OIL:**

This oil is obtained from the cummin seed, which is derived from the Nigella sativa tree/plant. This special oil intake has proven to drastically reduce or impede the growth of the H-pylori bacteria in the body. Its healing properties help in no small measure to heal/treat stomach lining ulcers.

⇘ **BROCCOLI SPROUTS:**

Studies have shown that eating broccoli sprouts freshly up to 80g or 100g every 24hrs for 60-80 days has reduced the amount of helicobacter pylori present in the individual's body very significantly.

FOODS TO AVOID WHEN HAVING H-PYLORI INFECTION.

Below is/are a list of foods to avoid when you happen to be a carrier of the H-pylori infection. Some of these foods include;

☞ COFFEE FOODS:

These are foods with high acidic content, and they can cause great discomfort and irritable effect on your stomach when you consume them. But if you must take them, it must be under the strict supervision or prescription of your health care expert.

➦ FRIED FOODS AND FOODS THAT CONTAINS FAT:

Foods that have a high amount of fatty content possess a large degree of oily content, and they take a longer digesting time than those that don't.

These meals require a greater amount of stomach acids to help with their digestion, and this digestion takes a long period to effectively be accomplished.

➦ SPICY AND PEPPERY FOODS:

Foods that contain excess pepper is/are a no for persons who are infected by H-pylori bacteria. This is because peppery foods contain a substance called capsaicin, which prompts the TRPV1 receptors, located in the upper gastric mucosa, which results in a very discomforting burning sensation.

⇘ <u>CHOCOLATE FOODS:</u>

These are foods that have theobromine and caffeine content in them. Caffeine obstructs the muscles that help to make a valve or an opening between the esophagus and the stomach of the human body. This could lead to muscular reflux, bearing in mind that caffeine and theobromine are more prominent in darker chocolates.

<u>SOME COMMON SIDE EFFECTS OF HELICOBACTER PYLORI TREATMENT.</u>

H-pylori medication just like some other diseases and infection treatments, comes with its peculiar side effects. However, these side effects aren't harmful to the body. Some of them include;

➫ <u>DIARRHEA:</u>

Diarrhea is also a common side effect of the treatment of Helicobacter pylori. Diarrhea occurs mainly due to the antibiotics that are used to treat the bacteria infection. To eliminate this side effect, eat easy digestibles like fish, drink a lot of yoghurt, and bring back to normal the intestinal flora of the stomach.

➫ <u>NAUSEA FEELING:</u>

This is a common H-pylori treatment side effect. Drink enough water to stay hydrated, eat crackers, and drink ginger tea and other easily digestibles, to eliminate this side effect.

↳ **METALLIC TASTE SENSATION IN THE TASTE BUDS:**

This is one of the most common after-medication side effects in the treatment of H-pylori. Never mind, it is not a major problem or something to be worried about. To eliminate this side effect, simply sprinkle salt on your toothbrush before brushing. This will help to neutralize the acidic content in the taste buds and also help in the production of more saliva in the mouth. You can make this a routine till you don't feel that sensation anymore.

CHAPTER EIGHT.

HELICOBACTER PYLORI TREATMENT PROCEDURES & SIDE-EFFECTS.

Just like every other ailment or disease, H -pylori can be treated. As earlier stated, H -pylori is a major cause of ulcers in the stomach linings of the body. Below are some of the possible treatment methods;

⇰ TREATING H-PYLORI WITH ANTIBIOTICS.

Studies have shown that antibiotics can treat Helicobacter pylori when prescribed and rightfully administered by certified medical experts. However, some recent studies have it that some types of H-pylori have proven resistant to antibiotic treatment.

This is by far the most common and widely used method for the treatment of H -pylori. Antibiotics could come in different forms (capsules or tablets).

Your certified health care professional will prescribe for you the best kind of antibiotics medicine that would best work for you in fighting the bacteria and keeping it away from you. However, below are some of the best and most widely used antibiotics in this context; Tetracycline, Amoxicillin Clarithromycin, Tinidazole, and Metronidazole.

✍ <u>TREATMENT WITH GARLIC FOODS.</u>

Garlic also is very rich in anti-bacterial and anti-inflammatory attributes. Both the anti-bacterial and anti-inflammatory features of garlic help to fight the H-pylori infection and as well alleviate the digestive system.

✍ <u>TREATMENT WITH GREEN TEA.</u>

This is a well-known anti-oxidant and anti-inflammatory food. The consumption of green tea can help to reduce the negative impact of H-pylori on the stomach wall lining. Green Derived from the herbal tea tree, green tea is another food substance that can help in reducing the H-pylori effect on individuals who suffer from the infection. This tea helps to prevent mucosal inflammation.

☙ <u>THE TRIPLE THERAPY (THE PROTON PUMP INHIBITORS TREATMENT).</u>

The double "P" and a "I" (PPI) treatment and combining them with two antibiotics treatment. This treatment plan or method must be under the strict supervision and monitoring of your healthcare expert.

The PPI therapy or treatment is an H-pylori treatment plan that helps to reduce the acidic content in the stomach, through the stalling of the small vessels that produce such acids. Some of these inhibitor drugs include; Omeprazole, Pantoprazole, Esomeprazole, and others.

From studies, it has been ascertained that there are currently two methods or kinds of Triple Therapy for the treatment of H - pylori. They are;

- ## **<u>The Rifabutioin Based Triple Therapy:</u>**

This treatment plan entails the use of two different kinds of antibiotics which could be rifabutin and amoxicillin taken with omeprazole. This medication mixture could be taken every 6 to 8 hours for two weeks.

- ## **<u>The clarithromycin Triple Therapy:</u>**

This medication comprises either Clarithromycin with Amoxicillin mixed with PPI or only Metronidazole mixed with PPI.

Medically, H-pylori-related ulcers often heal within a short period of weeks. It is advisable that you avoid NSAIDs drugs/medications such as ibuprofen and aspirin. Most medical experts may test you after a week or two of completion of your medication to ascertain total healing from the ailment.

➥ <u>THE BISMUTH SUBSALICYLATE TREATMENT METHOD.</u>

This treatment medication is often time used as a treatment for diarrhea. Administering this treatment method should be done with the close supervision of your health care expert.

➥ <u>THE HISTAMINE HINDERING THERAPY METHOD.</u>

This treatment seeks to hinder the histamine substance from creating or developing more acids in the stomach

CHAPTER NINE.

SIMPLE 7-DAY DIETARY PLAN, FOR H-PYLORI TREATMENT.

The adoption of a dietary plan for the treatment of H-pylori infection is a fundamental part of treating and managing the disease condition.

⧗ **DAY ONE:**

- *For Breakfast:* Eat some freshly plucked berries, mixed with honey and yoghurt blend.
- *For Lunch:* Eat fresh carrots, with meat and whole grain bread.
- *For Dinner:* Eat freshly prepared vegetable sauce with rice.

⧗ **DAY TWO:**

- ◆ *For Breakfast:* Take a cup of banana, milk, peanut butter, and spinach mixed smoothie flavor.
- ◆ *For Lunch:* Cucumber, tomatoes, and salad mixed with greens.
- ◆ *For Dinner:* Eat Asparagus, and cooked sweet potato.

⧖ **<u>DAY THREE:</u>**

- ◆ *For Breakfast:* Eat a whole grain meal, combined with some matted eggs.
- ◆ *For lunch:* Eat vegetables and grilled chicken.
- ◆ *For Dinner:* Take Veggies/greens, quinoa and some salmon.

⧖ **<u>DAY FOUR:</u>**

- *For Breakfast:* Eat matted eggs, avocado pear slice, and some fresh fruits.
- *For lunch:* Take some veggie soup, whole grain bread, and some toasted chicken
- For dinner: Eat some veggies and chicken breasts.

⧗ DAY FIVE:

- *For breakfast:* Take fresh berries, with whole grain biscuits.
- *For Lunch:* Eat Avocado pear, with grilled chicken, and greens.
- *For Dinner:* Take veggie sauce stew, some fresh fruits, and whole grain bread.

⧗ DAY SIX:

- ◆ *For Breakfast:* Take a cheese and veggie omelet, with whole grain rice.
- ◆ *For Lunch:* Eat Biscuits, some greens fruity, and tuna salad.
- ◆ *For Dinner:* Take Quinoa, baked root vegetables, and some pork meat.

⧖ **<u>DAY SEVEN:</u>**
- ◆ *For Breakfast:* Take some honey, Oats mixed with milk and some bananas.
- ◆ *For Lunch:* Fresh cherry tomatoes, well-grilled turkey or chicken breast, with cheese.
- ◆ *For Dinner:* Eat Roasted or cooked potatoes, some green beans, and some grilled shrimp.

CHAPTER TEN.

SOME HEALTHY PRACTICES TO KEEP AND FINAL THOUGHT.

Some healthy practices to keep that will aid your digestion:

As a result of the fact that H-pylori is a good reducing agent of stomach acids, which aids the body's digestion process(es), when a food substance is not well digested could result in nutrient deficiency, stomach bloating, fatigue, and constipation. Below are some easy-to-do things to help the digestion process;

- **Practice Frequent Eating:** Eating frequently but in small quantities, is a good way that will help hasten your digestion process. Consuming large meals could result in a slow digestion rate because it takes more time to digest large quantities of food.

- **<u>Practice Proper Chewing Of Food Before Swallowing:</u>** Since food chewing is the foremost step in the digestion process, it is best you choose your food very well in your mouth, before swallowing it/them. It is recommended that 5-10 chews should be the minimum number of chews before swallowing.

- **<u>Complete Your Meal Eating At The Table:</u>** When you eat, try to avoid the temptation of standing up and down, or taking breaks between a given meal before continuing the eating process. This could also result in a slow digestion process.

The bacteria virus itself is in a spiral circular plumpy nature. According to the

Centre for Disease Control, H-pylori affects over 2/3 of the population of the world.

THE END!

www.ingramcontent.com/pod-product-compliance
Lightning Source LLC
Chambersburg PA
CBHW071549260726
48653CB00007BA/2579